Arthritis-Free Aging

Complete Guide to Joint Health and Pain-free Living for Seniors

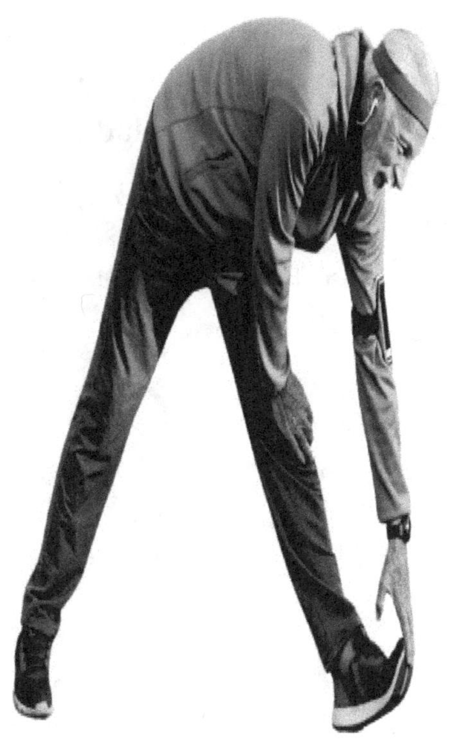

Jack Randy

Table of Contents

INTRODUCTION

Meet Thompson, a lively senior who loved spending his retirement years exploring the world. However, arthritis had started to creep into his life, bringing pain and discomfort that threatened his adventures. His mobility and flexibility dwindled as the condition advanced, and he grew concerned about falling, which would shatter his independence.

One day, Thompson's daughter introduced him to a book called "Arthritis-Free Aging." Skeptical but willing to try anything, Thompson began following the advice within the pages. As he delved into the book, he discovered a wealth of information about managing arthritis, easing pain, and regaining his mobility. Thompson started incorporating arthritis-friendly exercises and joint-strengthening routines into his daily life. Slowly but surely, he felt the difference. The pain became less of a constant companion, and his once-stiff joints started to regain their flexibility.

With newfound strength and balance, Thompson's confidence soared. The fall prevention tips he learned became invaluable, allowing him to continue exploring the world with less fear of accidents. Thanks to the "Arthritis-Free Aging" book, Thompson's golden years became vibrant and pain-free. His days were once again filled with travel, laughter, and cherished moments, proving that with the right knowledge and dedication, arthritis can be managed, and life can be lived to the fullest.

CHAPTER ONE

UNDERSTANDING ARTHRITIS

Arthritis simply refers to a group of joint disorders characterized by inflammation and pain that can limit mobility and affect the quality of life, especially in aging individuals. This book addresses various forms of arthritis, emphasizing methods to manage, prevent, and alleviate its symptoms, allowing seniors to enjoy pain-free and mobile aging. Through exercise, lifestyle adjustments, and fall prevention techniques, the goal is to help aging individuals combat arthritis and promote an active, independent, and fulfilling life.

Types Of Arthritis In Seniors

Arthritis in seniors encompasses a range of types, each with its characteristics and challenges. The most prevalent forms affecting older individuals include:

Osteoarthritis (OA): Often referred to as "wear and tear" arthritis, OA is the most common type. It results from the gradual deterioration of cartilage, leading to joint pain, stiffness, and reduced mobility. Seniors may experience OA in weight-bearing joints like the hips, knees, and spine.

Rheumatoid Arthritis (RA): This is an autoimmune disease where the body's immune system mistakenly attacks healthy joint tissues. RA can affect any joint, leading to pain, swelling, and even joint deformities.

Gout: Gout is caused by the accumulation of uric acid crystals in the joints, often in the big toe. It results in sudden and severe pain, redness, and swelling.

Psoriatic Arthritis: This type of arthritis typically affects individuals with psoriasis, a skin condition. It causes joint pain, stiffness, and swelling, often in the fingers and toes.

Ankylosing Spondylitis: This chronic inflammatory condition primarily targets the spine and can cause pain and stiffness, especially in the lower back and hips.

Juvenile Arthritis: While not exclusive to seniors, some individuals may continue to experience arthritis symptoms that originated in their childhood.

Understanding the specific type of arthritis an older individual is dealing with is crucial for effective management and treatment. "Arthritis-Free Aging" provides guidance and exercises tailored to various arthritis types to help seniors maintain mobility, alleviate pain, and enjoy a higher quality of life in their later years.

Impact Of Arthritis On Aging

Arthritis has a profound impact on the aging population, affecting their overall quality of life and daily activities. Several key factors illustrate the significant influence of arthritis on seniors:

Pain and Discomfort: Arthritis commonly causes pain, stiffness, and joint swelling, making even simple tasks like walking, dressing, or climbing stairs challenging. Persistent pain can lead to fatigue, decreased mobility, and reduced participation in social and recreational activities.

Reduced Mobility: One of the most noticeable consequences of arthritis is the decline in mobility and flexibility. As seniors struggle with joint discomfort, they become more sedentary, which can lead to muscle weakness, further limiting their ability to move freely.

Depression and Anxiety: The chronic pain and disability associated with arthritis can contribute to mental health issues, such as depression and anxiety. Seniors may experience frustration and emotional distress due to the limitations placed on their daily lives.

Decreased Independence: Arthritis can challenge seniors' independence, as they may require assistance with daily activities they once managed on their own. This increased reliance on caregivers or family members can be emotionally taxing.

Increased Fall Risk: Seniors with arthritis are at a higher risk of falls due to balance issues and joint pain. Falls can lead to serious injuries, further reducing their independence and overall well-being.

Common Symptoms And Signs Of Arthritis In Seniors

Common symptoms and signs of arthritis in seniors include joint pain, stiffness, and swelling. Seniors with arthritis may experience reduced range of motion, making it difficult to move joints freely. Morning stiffness is a typical complaint, as joints take time to loosen up. Arthritis can lead to deformities, such as knobby finger joints or joint misalignment. Fatigue and muscle weakness are common, often affecting mobility and leading to a sedentary lifestyle. Additionally, seniors may notice redness or warmth around affected joints. Understanding these symptoms is crucial for early diagnosis and effective management of arthritis, improving the quality of life for older individuals.

Diagnosing Arthritis

Diagnosing arthritis is a critical step in the journey to arthritis-free aging. Medical professionals utilize various methods to identify arthritis in seniors. Clinical assessment and patient history play a fundamental role, as seniors often describe their symptoms and medical history. Imaging techniques like X-rays and MRIs offer visual confirmation of joint damage, cartilage deterioration, and other structural abnormalities.

Blood tests may detect specific markers like C-reactive protein and rheumatoid factor, indicative of certain arthritis types, such as rheumatoid arthritis. Joint fluid analysis, involving the extraction of synovial fluid from an affected joint, can help diagnose conditions like gout.

Additionally, physical examinations assess joint tenderness, swelling, and range of motion. Combining these approaches allows healthcare providers to determine the type of arthritis and develop personalized strategies for managing the condition. Timely and accurate diagnosis is crucial for implementing the right interventions, ensuring arthritis doesn't limit seniors' quality of life and overall well-being in their aging journey.

Understanding Arthritis Triggers

Understanding arthritis triggers is essential for managing and preventing arthritis-related issues in seniors. Arthritis symptoms can be triggered by various factors, including:

Diet and Nutrition: Certain foods, particularly those high in purines, can exacerbate gout, while an anti-inflammatory diet can help reduce arthritis symptoms.

Weight Management: Excess weight adds stress to the joints, particularly those in the lower body, increasing the risk and severity of arthritis.

Physical Activity: Regular, appropriate exercise can strengthen muscles, support joint health, and prevent stiffness. However, overexertion or inadequate exercise can lead to joint problems.

Environmental Factors: Changes in temperature, humidity, and atmospheric pressure can influence arthritis symptoms, causing flares.

Infections and Injuries: Infections can trigger inflammatory arthritis, while joint injuries or overuse can lead to osteoarthritis.

Stress and Mental Health: Emotional stress can exacerbate arthritis symptoms, so maintaining mental well-being is vital.

By recognizing these triggers, seniors can take proactive steps to minimize their impact, such as maintaining a healthy diet, staying physically active, managing stress, and being cautious in challenging environments. This understanding empowers seniors in their journey toward arthritis-free aging.

CHAPTER TWO

CAUSES AND RISK FACTORS

The Role Of Age In Arthritis

The role of age in arthritis is significant, as it is a condition that predominantly affects seniors. Arthritis becomes more prevalent and often more severe with advancing age. There are several important components to this interaction.

Cartilage Wear and Tear: Over time, the cartilage that cushions joints naturally wears down. This age-related process can lead to osteoarthritis, the most common type of arthritis in older adults.

Joint Overuse: Years of use can take a toll on joints. Occupations or activities that require repetitive joint movement or excessive stress can contribute to arthritis.

Weakening Immune System: As individuals age, their immune systems may become less effective at maintaining proper immune responses. This can lead to autoimmune forms of arthritis.

Genetic Predisposition: Some forms of arthritis have genetic links, and these may become more apparent as individuals age.

Comorbidity: Aging often brings additional health concerns like obesity, diabetes, and cardiovascular issues, which can exacerbate arthritis symptoms.

While arthritis is more common in older individuals, it's important to note that it's not an inevitable part of aging. Seniors can take proactive steps to manage arthritis and maintain joint health, focusing on nutrition, exercise, and lifestyle modifications to lead an active and pain-free life.

Genetics And Arthritis

Genetics plays a significant role in arthritis, particularly in the context of arthritis-free aging. Certain forms of arthritis, like rheumatoid arthritis, have a strong genetic component. Individuals with a family history of arthritis are at a higher risk of developing the condition, underscoring the genetic influence.

Genetic factors can determine a person's susceptibility to arthritis triggers and the severity of their symptoms. However, while genetics may increase the likelihood of arthritis, it's not the sole determinant.

Lifestyle, environmental factors, and aging also contribute. Arthritis-free aging focuses on understanding genetic predispositions and leveraging lifestyle changes to minimize the impact of these genetic influences, helping individuals maintain joint health and mobility as they age.

Lifestyle Factors And Arthritis

Lifestyle factors play a crucial role in arthritis, a focal point in arthritis-free aging. Certain lifestyle choices can either exacerbate or alleviate arthritis symptoms. Sedentary habits and poor dietary choices can contribute to weight gain, which places excess stress on joints. In contrast, regular physical activity, especially arthritis-specific exercises, helps improve joint flexibility and reduce pain.

Additionally, a balanced diet rich in anti-inflammatory foods can combat inflammation associated with arthritis. Smoking and excessive alcohol consumption are lifestyle factors that can worsen arthritis symptoms. Arthritis-free aging encourages seniors to make positive lifestyle changes by adopting a physically active routine, maintaining a healthy diet, and avoiding harmful habits to reduce the impact of arthritis and promote a more pain-free, mobile, and active life.

Joint Injuries And Arthritis Development

Joint injuries can significantly contribute to the development of arthritis, a key concern addressed in arthritis-free aging. When an injury occurs, such as a sprain, fracture, or ligament tear, it can disrupt the natural alignment and function of the affected joint. Even after the injury heals, the joint may remain vulnerable.

Post-injury, the joint might not move as efficiently, causing uneven stress and potential damage to cartilage and surrounding tissues. These injuries trigger the release of inflammatory chemicals that can lead to chronic inflammation and long-term damage, a primary factor in arthritis development.

For seniors, who may have a history of joint injuries from sports, accidents, or repetitive motions in their younger years, addressing these injuries and their associated inflammation is essential in preventing or managing arthritis. The arthritis-free aging approach emphasizes joint care, including proper rehabilitation after injury, to reduce the risk of arthritis.

The Connection Between Inflammation And Arthritis

Inflammation is a central element in the development and progression of arthritis, a critical aspect explored in arthritis-free aging. Arthritis refers to a group of inflammatory joint disorders, and inflammation plays a fundamental role in most types of arthritis. When the body's immune system mistakenly activates an inflammatory response in the joints, it can lead to chronic inflammation, which, over time, damages cartilage, bones, and surrounding tissues.

Inflammation contributes to pain, swelling, and stiffness in the affected joints, reducing mobility and diminishing the overall quality of life, especially for seniors. As the inflammation persists, it accelerates joint deterioration. This link between inflammation and arthritis underscores the importance of addressing inflammation through lifestyle, dietary choices, and exercise, as emphasized in arthritis-free aging. Seniors can adopt strategies to manage inflammation effectively, reduce arthritis symptoms, and promote joint health, enhancing their overall well-being.

CHAPTER THREE

PREVENTING ARTHRITIS IN SENIORS

Diet And Nutrition For Joint Health

Diet and nutrition play a crucial role in maintaining joint health and preventing arthritis in seniors. A well-balanced diet provides essential nutrients that support joint function, reduce inflammation, and slow down the progression of arthritis.

A diet rich in antioxidants, such as vitamins C and E, can help protect joints from damage caused by free radicals. Omega-3 fatty acids, found in fatty fish like salmon and walnuts, have anti-inflammatory properties that can alleviate arthritis symptoms.

Additionally, consuming foods high in fiber, like whole grains and plenty of fruits and vegetables, can help control weight, which is essential for reducing stress on joints.

Seniors should aim to maintain a healthy body weight as excess weight places added strain on joints, especially the knees and hips. Achieving and sustaining a healthy weight through proper diet and exercise can significantly reduce the risk of developing arthritis or alleviate its symptoms in those who already have it.

Maintaining A Healthy Weight

Maintaining a healthy weight is a critical component of preventing arthritis in seniors. Excess weight places increased stress on joints, especially in weight-bearing areas like the knees and hips. This extra pressure can accelerate joint degeneration and increase the risk of developing arthritis or exacerbate its symptoms.

Adopting a lifestyle that includes a balanced diet and regular exercise helps seniors achieve and maintain a healthy weight. Proper weight management not only lessens the load on joints but also reduces inflammation, a key contributor to arthritis. Seniors can work with healthcare professionals to create personalized weight management plans that fit their specific needs, contributing to a healthier, arthritis-free aging journey.

Exercise And Physical Activity

Exercise and physical activity play a pivotal role in preventing arthritis among seniors. Regular physical activity helps maintain joint flexibility, strength, and overall health.

It can also aid in weight management, reducing the strain on joints, and combat inflammation.

Engaging in exercises that promote joint mobility and muscle strength, such as walking, swimming, or yoga, can significantly contribute to arthritis prevention. Seniors should aim for a well-rounded fitness routine to ensure their bodies remain strong, flexible, and less susceptible to the development of arthritis. Staying active not only enhances joint health but also supports overall well-being as seniors age gracefully.

Joint Protection Techniques

Joint protection techniques are essential for preventing arthritis in seniors. These strategies help safeguard the joints, reduce the risk of inflammation, and maintain their overall function. Here are several important techniques to consider:

Proper Ergonomics: Maintaining good posture and using ergonomic tools can reduce strain on the joints, especially in daily activities.

Weight Management: Maintaining a healthy weight alleviates excess stress on the joints, particularly those of the knees, hips, and lower back.

Regular Exercise: Engaging in low-impact exercises, such as swimming, walking, and cycling, helps to strengthen muscles around the joints, enhancing support and reducing wear and tear.

Balanced Nutrition: A diet rich in anti-inflammatory foods, such as fruits, vegetables, and omega-3 fatty acids, can aid in joint health.

Protective Gear: Seniors involved in activities that place stress on their joints should use appropriate protective gear, like knee braces or wrist supports.

Proper Lifting Techniques: Utilizing proper body mechanics when lifting heavy objects minimizes the risk of joint injury, particularly in the spine and back.

Joint-Friendly Activities: Seniors should focus on exercises and activities that are gentle on the joints, avoiding high-impact sports that can lead to joint strain.

By following these joint protection techniques, seniors can reduce the likelihood of arthritis and enjoy greater joint health as they age.

Medication and Supplements for Prevention

Medications and supplements can play a crucial role in the prevention of arthritis in seniors. While they are not a guaranteed shield against this condition, they can help reduce inflammation, ease pain, and support overall joint health. Here are some options to consider:

Anti-Inflammatory Medications: Non-steroidal anti-inflammatory drugs (NSAIDs) can help manage inflammation and provide relief from arthritis symptoms. However, their long-term use should be monitored by a healthcare professional.

Disease-Modifying Antirheumatic Drugs (DMARDs): In some cases, especially with rheumatoid arthritis, DMARDs can slow down the progression of the disease and protect the joints from further damage.

Corticosteroids: These anti-inflammatory medications can be used to manage severe arthritis symptoms and provide short-term relief.

Joint Supplements: Glucosamine and chondroitin sulfate are commonly taken by seniors to support joint health. These supplements may help maintain cartilage and reduce pain.

Vitamins and Minerals: Nutritional supplements like vitamin D and calcium can aid in bone health, which is closely linked to joint health.

Dietary Changes: A balanced diet that includes anti-inflammatory foods like turmeric, ginger, and omega-3 fatty acids can reduce inflammation and protect the joints.

It's crucial for seniors to consult with a healthcare provider before starting any medication or supplement regimen. The choice of intervention should be based on an individual's health status and specific arthritis risk factors. A healthcare professional can provide personalized guidance to help seniors navigate the most suitable approach to prevent arthritis.

CHAPTER FOUR

SIMPLE EXERCISES FOR ARTHRITIS-FREE AGING

Warm-Up exercises

1. Neck Tilts:

Introduction: Neck tilts are essential to improve neck flexibility and reduce stiffness.

Instructions:

1. Sit or stand up straight.

2. Tilt your head slightly to the side, bringing your ear close to your shoulder.

3. Hold for 15-20 seconds.

4. Return to the starting position.

5. Repeat on the other side.

Sets and Repetitions: 2 sets of 5 repetitions on each side.

2. Shoulder Rolls:

Introduction: Shoulder rolls help to warm up and improve mobility in the shoulder joints.

Instructions:

1. Stand or sit with your arms relaxed at your sides.
2. Slowly roll your shoulders in a circular motion, moving them forward, up, back, and down.
3. Complete 10-12 rolls in one direction.
4. Then, reverse the direction.

Sets and Repetitions: 2 sets of 10-12 rolls in each direction.

3. Arm Swings:

Introduction*:* Arm swings enhance blood circulation to the arms and shoulders, reducing the risk of arthritis-related discomfort.

Instructions*:*

1. Stand with your feet shoulder-width apart.
2. Swing your arms forward and backward in a controlled, rhythmic motion.
3. Keep your arms relaxed and extended.
4. Perform for 30 seconds.

Sets and Repetitions*:* 2 sets of 30 seconds.

4. Hip Circles:

Introduction*:* Hip circles improve hip joint flexibility and reduce stiffness in the lower back.

Instructions*:*

1. Stand with your hands on your hips.

2. Make circular motions with your hips, moving them forward, to the side, back, and to the other side.

3. Perform 10-12 circles in one direction.

4. Then, switch to the opposite direction.

Sets and Repetitions: 2 sets of 10-12 circles in each direction.

5. Ankle Pumps:

Introduction: Ankle pumps are excellent for warming up the ankle joints and promoting better circulation in the lower extremities.

Instructions:

1. Maintain a flat foot position while sitting.

2. Lift your toes off the ground while keeping your heels on the floor.

3. Lower your toes back down.

4. Repeat this pumping motion.

5. Perform for 20 seconds.

Sets and Repetitions*:* 2 sets of 20 seconds.

These warm-up exercises are designed to prepare the body for more extensive physical activity. Seniors should perform these exercises gently, without pushing their joints too far. The goal is to increase blood flow, improve flexibility, and reduce the risk of injury, promoting arthritis-free aging.

Stretching Exercises

1. Neck Stretch:

Introduction*:* Neck stretches are essential to improve neck flexibility, reduce tension, and relieve neck pain.

Instructions*:*

1. Sit or stand with your back straight.

2. Slowly tilt your head to one side, bringing your ear toward your shoulder.

3. Hold the stretch for 15-20 seconds.

4. Return to the starting position.

5. Repeat on the other side.

Sets and Repetitions: 2 sets of 2 stretches on each side.

2. Shoulder Stretch:

Introduction: Shoulder stretches help improve shoulder mobility and reduce discomfort in the upper body.

Instructions:

1. Stand or sit with your back straight.

2. Extend one arm across your chest.

3. Use the opposite hand to gently press the extended arm closer to your chest.

4. Hold the stretch for 20-30 seconds.

5. Switch to the other arm.

Sets and Repetitions: 2 sets of 1 stretch on each arm.

3. Hip Flexor Stretch:

Introduction: Hip flexor stretches are beneficial for improving hip mobility and relieving lower back pain.

Instructions:

1. Place one foot in front of you and the other behind you.

2. Your back leg should remain straight while you bend your front knee.

3. Gently push your hips forward.

4. Hold for 20-30 seconds.

5. Switch to the other leg.

Sets and Repetitions: 2 sets of 1 stretch on each leg.

4. Quadriceps Stretch:

Introduction: Quadriceps stretches help maintain flexibility in the thigh muscles, reducing stress on the knee joints.

Instructions:

1. Stand on one leg while holding onto a stable surface for balance.

2. Bend your other leg and grab your ankle behind you.

3. Gently pull your ankle towards your buttocks.

4. Hold for 20-30 seconds.

5. Switch to the other leg.

Sets and Repetitions: 2 sets of 1 stretch on each leg.

5. Calf Stretch:

Introduction: Calf stretches promote calf muscle flexibility and help reduce the risk of ankle and calf pain.

Instructions:

1. Put your hands against a wall while facing it.

2. As you take a step back, set your heel firmly on the ground.

3. Lean forward to feel the stretch in your calf.

4. Hold for 20-30 seconds.

5. Switch to the other leg.

Sets and Repetitions: 2 sets of 1 stretch on each leg.

These stretching exercises are designed to increase flexibility, reduce tension, and promote joint health. Seniors should perform these stretches gently and avoid overstretching, especially if they have arthritis. Stretching helps maintain a full range of motion and reduces the risk of joint stiffness and pain.

Low-impact Aerobic

1. Walking:

Introduction: Walking is a low-impact aerobic exercise that enhances cardiovascular health and maintains joint mobility.

Instructions:

1. Find a level, comfortable surface to walk on.

2. Start with a slow, steady pace.

3. Walk for 15-20 minutes, gradually increasing the duration as your fitness improves.

Sets and Repetitions: Aim for 3-5 times a week.

2. Swimming:

Introduction: Swimming is an excellent choice for seniors, as it's easy on the joints while providing a full-body workout.

Instructions:

1. Visit a local pool with a lifeguard.

2. Engage in a gentle swim for 20-30 minutes.

3. Gradually increase your swimming duration.

Sets and Repetitions: Aim for 2-3 times a week.

3. Stationary Cycling:

Introduction: Stationary cycling is a low-impact aerobic exercise that improves leg strength and cardiovascular fitness.

Instructions:

1. Use a stationary bike at home or a fitness center.
2. Start with 10-15 minutes of cycling.
3. Increase your cycling time as you become more comfortable.

Sets and Repetitions: Aim for 3-5 times a week.

4. Seated Marching:

Introduction: Seated marching is a safe, low-impact exercise that can be done while sitting in a sturdy chair.

Instructions:

1. Sit up straight in a chair.

2. Lift one knee as high as comfortable while keeping the other foot flat on the floor.

3. Alternate legs in a marching motion.

4. Continue for 5-10 minutes.

Sets and Repetitions: Perform this exercise as needed throughout the day.

5. Tai Chi:

Introduction: Tai Chi is a gentle, low-impact martial art that focuses on balance, flexibility, and mental well-being.

Instructions:

1. Enroll in a Tai Chi class or use online resources.

2. Follow the instructor's movements, focusing on controlled, flowing motions.

3. Start with 15-20 minutes of Tai Chi practice.

Sets and Repetitions: Aim for 2-3 times a week.

Low-impact aerobic exercises like these help seniors maintain cardiovascular fitness, joint mobility, and overall well-being while minimizing the risk of stress on arthritic joints. As with any exercise program, it's essential to consult a healthcare provider or fitness professional before starting a new routine, especially if you have arthritis.

Strengthening Exercises For Joints And Muscles

1. Leg Raises:

Introduction: Leg raises are ideal for strengthening the muscles in your thighs and hips, improving balance and stability.

Instructions:

1. For support, take a seat next to a strong chair.

2. Lift one leg straight out to the side.

3. Lower it back down and repeat.

Perform 2 sets of 10 repetitions on each leg.

2. Wall Push-Ups:

Introduction: Wall push-ups are an excellent upper body strengthener without the strain of traditional push-ups.

Instructions:

1. Stand facing a wall at arm's length.

2. Hold the wall with your hands at shoulder height.

3. Bend your elbows and lean toward the wall.

4. Push back to the starting position.

Perform 2 sets of 10 repetitions.

3. Seated Knee Extensions:

Introduction: Seated knee extensions target the quadriceps muscles to help maintain strong, stable knees.

Instructions:

1. Sit up straight in a sturdy chair with your feet flat on the floor.

2. Extend one leg straight out, and hold for a few seconds.

3. Return to the starting position.

Perform 2 sets of 10 repetitions for each leg.

4. Bicep Curls:

Introduction: Bicep curls strengthen the muscles in your arms and improve your ability to lift and carry objects.

Instructions:

1. Sit in a chair with a dumbbell or a household item in each hand.

2. Keep your back straight and your arms hanging at your sides.

3. Curl the weights up toward your chest.

4. Lower them back down.

Perform 2 sets of 10 repetitions for each arm.

5. Standing Heel Raises:

Introduction: Standing heel raises are great for calf muscle strength and balance, helping to prevent falls.

Instructions:

1. Stand behind a chair or counter for support.

2. Slowly raise your heels off the ground as high as you can.

3. Lower them back down.

Perform 2 sets of 10 repetitions.

Strengthening exercises like these can enhance joint support, maintain muscle mass, and reduce the risk of falls, which are critical aspects of Arthritis-free Aging. Always remember to consult with a healthcare provider or fitness professional before starting a new exercise routine, especially if you have arthritis or any underlying health concerns.

Balance And Coordination Exercises

1. Single-Leg Balance:

Introduction: Single-leg balance exercises are crucial for improving stability and preventing falls.

Instructions:

1. Stand next to a sturdy chair or counter for support.

2. Lift one foot slightly off the ground and balance on the other.

3. Hold for 20-30 seconds.

4. Switch legs and repeat.

Perform 2 sets for each leg.

2. Tandem Walk:

Introduction: Tandem walking challenges your balance and coordination.

Instructions:

1. Find a clear, open space.

2. Take small, deliberate steps, placing one foot directly in front of the other.

3. Walk forward for about 10 steps.

4. Turn around and walk back.

Perform 2 sets.

3. Heel-to-Toe Walk:

Introduction: Heel-to-toe walking mimics the sobriety test and enhances balance and coordination.

Instructions:

1. Stand with your feet touching.
2. Take a step forward with one foot, placing the heel of the front foot against the toes of the back foot.
3. Continue with a heel-to-toe pattern for about 10 steps.
4. Turn around and walk back.

Perform 2 sets.

4. Clock Reach:

Introduction: The clock reach exercise challenges your balance by reaching in different directions.

Instructions:

1. Stand with a chair in front of you.

2. Imagine yourself at the center of a clock.

3. Reach your right hand to 12 o'clock, then 3 o'clock, 6 o'clock, and 9 o'clock.

4. Perform the same sequence with your left hand.

Perform 2 sets in each direction.

5. Ball Catch and Toss:

Introduction*:* This exercise combines hand-eye coordination and balance skills.

Instructions*:*

1. Stand with your feet shoulder-width apart.

2. Have a partner (or a wall) gently toss a softball to you.

3. Catch and toss the ball back.

4. Repeat for 2-3 minutes.

Perform 2 sets.

Balance and coordination exercises like these can help enhance stability, reduce the risk of falls, and improve overall mobility, all essential components of Arthritis-free Aging.

Flexibility And Range Of Motion Exercises

1. Spinal Twist:

Introduction*:* Spinal twists promote spinal flexibility and alleviate lower back discomfort.

Instructions*:*

1. Place your feet flat on the floor while you sit on a chair.

2. For stability, grab onto the chair's back.

3. Turn your upper body slightly to one side.

4. Hold for 15-20 seconds.

5. Return to the center and repeat on the other side.

Perform 2 sets for each side.

2. Wrist Flexor and Extensor Stretch:

Introduction: This exercise helps improve wrist flexibility and reduce discomfort associated with arthritis.

Instructions:

1. Extend one arm forward with your palm facing up.

2. Use your opposite hand to gently pull your fingers back.

3. Hold for 15-20 seconds.

4. Turn your wrist so that the palm is facing down.

5. Use your opposite hand to gently push your fingers back.

6. Hold for 15-20 seconds.

7. Repeat with the other arm.

Perform 2 sets for each wrist.

3. Trunk Rotation:

Introduction: Trunk rotations improve spinal flexibility and reduce lower back discomfort.

Instructions:

1. Sit on a chair with your feet flat on the floor.

2. Keep your hips and knees facing forward.

3. Slowly rotate your upper body to one side.

4. Hold for 15-20 seconds.

5. Return to the center and repeat on the other side.

Perform 2 sets for each side.

4. Hip Flexor Stretch:
Introduction: Hip flexor stretches help maintain hip flexibility and improve posture.

Instructions:
1. Stand with your feet hip-width apart.
2. Take a step back with one foot.
3. Bend the front knee and gently push your hips forward.
4. Hold for 15-20 seconds.
5. Repeat with the other leg.

Perform 2 sets for each leg.

5. Ankle Circles:

Introduction: Ankle circles enhance ankle flexibility, helping with balance and mobility.

Instructions:

1. Sit on a chair with your feet flat on the floor.
2. Lift one foot slightly off the ground.
3. Turn your ankle clockwise and then anticlockwise in a circular manner.
4. Complete 10 circles for each direction. Repeat with the other ankle.

Perform 2 sets for each ankle.

Flexibility and range of motion exercises like these can help alleviate stiffness, improve posture, and enhance overall mobility, contributing to Arthritis-free Aging.

CHAPTER FIVE

DAILY LIFESTYLE HABITS FOR JOINT HEALTH

Ergonomics in Everyday Life

Ergonomics plays a vital role in promoting joint health and overall well-being in our daily lives. It's the science of designing and arranging our environments to fit the individuals who use them, to reduce stress on the body. In the context of daily lifestyle habits for joint health, incorporating ergonomics means making mindful choices to minimize strain on the joints and maximize comfort.

For example, when working at a desk, ensuring the height and position of your chair, keyboard, and monitor are ergonomically aligned can prevent neck, back, and wrist discomfort. When lifting objects, using proper lifting techniques and tools can protect the joints, particularly the spine and knees.

Ergonomics extends to all aspects of life, from the way we sit, stand, and move to the tools and equipment we use. By paying attention to ergonomics, individuals can significantly reduce the risk of joint stress, strain, and the development of arthritis or related conditions. These simple adjustments can lead to a healthier, more comfortable, and more joint-friendly daily life.

Home Modifications For Arthritis Relief

Home modifications can be a game-changer for individuals dealing with arthritis. Simple changes to the living environment can provide significant relief for sore and aching joints. This includes installing handrails in key areas like bathrooms and staircases, reducing the need to strain joints during daily activities. Additionally, replacing traditional doorknobs with lever-style handles, which require less force to operate, eases hand and wrist pain.

For kitchens, using pull-out shelves and drawers minimizes bending and stretching, reducing stress on knee and hip joints. Raised toilet seats and shower chairs improve bathroom accessibility and safety. Finally, adding cushioning to chairs and beds can enhance comfort and reduce joint pain, making home life more manageable for those with arthritis.

Stress Reduction Techniques

Stress is not only a mental burden but can also manifest physically and exacerbate the symptoms of arthritis. To manage joint health effectively, incorporating stress reduction techniques into your daily routine is crucial. Engaging in relaxation practices, such as meditation, deep breathing, or mindfulness, can help soothe both the mind and the body. These techniques can reduce muscle tension and joint inflammation, providing much-needed relief.

Regular physical activity, in the form of gentle exercises like yoga or tai chi, can contribute to stress reduction while promoting flexibility and balance. Adequate sleep is equally vital, as it allows your body to repair and rejuvenate, supporting overall joint health.

Prioritizing time for hobbies, socializing, and relaxation can help combat stress and contribute to a more balanced, joint-friendly lifestyle. Reducing stress might not be a direct cure for arthritis, but it can significantly improve the quality of life for those affected by this condition.

Staying Active And Engaged

Maintaining an active and engaged lifestyle is pivotal in preserving joint health for aging individuals. Regular physical activity helps keep joints supple and minimizes stiffness, which is particularly vital for those with or at risk of arthritis. Engaging in low-impact exercises like walking, swimming, or cycling can improve flexibility and strengthen the muscles that support the joints.

Additionally, participating in social activities and hobbies can contribute to overall well-being and a healthier outlook. Staying connected with friends and family not only provides emotional support but also encourages participation in various activities, which can be particularly beneficial in warding off arthritis symptoms.

An active and engaged lifestyle may also involve volunteering, learning new skills, or pursuing interests and passions. This not only keeps the mind sharp but also provides a sense of purpose and fulfillment. In summary, staying active and engaged is a holistic approach to joint health that benefits both the body and the spirit.

7-DAY EXERCISE PLAN

Day 1: Warm-Up

Exercise: Ankle Pumps

Instructions: While seated, lift one foot, point your toes up and down.

Sets: 2

Repetitions: 10 on each foot

Day 2: Stretching

Exercise: Neck Stretch

Instructions: Gently tilt your head to one side, holding for 10 seconds.

Sets: 2

Repetitions: 3 on each side

Day 3: Low-Impact Aerobics

Exercise: Stationary Cycling (if available)

Instructions: Pedal at a comfortable pace while seated.

Time: 15 minutes

Day 4: Strengthening

Exercise: Seated Leg Raise

Instructions: While seated, straighten one leg and hold for 5 seconds.

Sets: 3

Repetitions: 10 on each leg

Day 5: Balance and Coordination

Exercise: Heel-to-Toe Walk

Instructions: Walk in a straight line, placing your heel in front of your toe with each step.

Sets: 2

Repetitions: 10 steps forward and 10 steps backward

Day 6: Flexibility and Range of Motion

Exercise: Shoulder Stretch
Instructions: Gently pull one arm across your chest and hold for 10 seconds.

Sets: 2

Repetitions: 3 on each arm

Day 7: Full-Body Workout

Exercise: Chair Squats
Instructions: Stand up from a chair, then sit back down without using your hands.

Sets: 3

Repetitions: 10

Remember to listen to your body, and if an exercise causes pain or discomfort, stop and consult with a healthcare professional. This 7-Day Exercise Plan aims to improve mobility, reduce pain, and enhance joint health. Regular exercise, combined with the other strategies discussed in the book, will pave the way for Arthritis-free Aging.

CONCLUSION

In concluding this journey towards Arthritis-free Aging, it's crucial to reflect on the incredible impact that making the right choices can have on our lives. The road to healthier, more flexible joints may seem daunting, but the effort is undoubtedly worthwhile. Throughout this book, we've explored the various facets of arthritis, from its types and diagnosis to the essential strategies for prevention and relief. We've understood how factors like genetics, lifestyle, and injuries play a pivotal role in its development. We've discovered the significance of a balanced diet, maintaining a healthy weight, and incorporating regular exercise into our daily routines. These are not merely guidelines but life-changing tools.

Each of you, dear readers, has the power to overcome the challenges posed by arthritis. Whether you're seeking prevention, relief, or improvement in your joint health, the answers lie within these pages. Your future of mobility, freedom from pain, and a fulfilling life are now firmly within your grasp.

Embrace the positive changes suggested within these chapters. Start with small, manageable steps and watch them grow into lifelong habits. Make the decision to take control of your health, ensure a pain-free future, and relish the independence that comes with it. Don't let arthritis dictate your path. Together, let's unlock the potential for an active, pain-free life that arthritis should never deny you. It's never too late to begin, and you are never too old to make a difference in your life. The journey towards

Arthritis-free Aging starts now. Commit to it. Embrace it. And experience the transformation it brings to your life, your joints, and your well-being. Your healthier, more active future awaits – seize it with confidence, determination, and a renewed zest for life.